The Monthly Switch
31 Essential Oil Recipes to Change Your Makeup Bag

LUCY NEWTON

ISBN: 9798332168895

DEDICATION

To my Husband and Children, Adam, Phoebe, Tommy & Minnie, thank you for always believing in me..

CONTENTS

1. INTRODUCTION

In a world increasingly aware of health and environmental impacts, many people are turning to natural alternatives in all areas of their lives, including their beauty regimes. Traditional beauty products, often laden with synthetic chemicals and artificial ingredients, are being swapped out for natural, plant-based solutions. This shift is more than just a trend; it's a movement toward holistic well-being, environmental sustainability, and a more conscious way of living.

Conventional beauty products can contain a myriad of chemicals, some of which have been linked to various health issues. Ingredients like parabens, phthalates, sulfates, and synthetic fragrances can disrupt the endocrine system, cause skin irritation, and even contribute to long-term health problems such as hormone imbalance and cancer. These substances can also have detrimental effects on the environment, contaminating water sources and harming wildlife.

Swapping chemical-laden beauty products for natural alternatives offers numerous benefits for your health, your skin, and the planet. Natural ingredients like essential oils, shea butter, and aloe vera are packed with vitamins, antioxidants, and nutrients that nourish the skin. These ingredients promote healthy skin function and repair, leading to a more radiant and youthful complexion. Synthetic chemicals can irritate the skin, causing redness, dryness, and allergic reactions. Natural products, on the other hand, are generally gentler and less likely to cause irritation, making them suitable for all skin types, including sensitive skin.

Moreover, essential oils offer therapeutic benefits. Lavender oil can help with relaxation and sleep, tea tree oil has antibacterial properties, and peppermint oil can invigorate and refresh. Incorporating these oils into your beauty routine can enhance both your physical and mental well-being. Reducing your exposure to harmful chemicals can have a positive impact on your overall health. By choosing natural beauty products, you are making a conscious decision to protect your body from potential toxins.

Natural beauty products often use sustainably sourced ingredients that are biodegradable and less harmful to the environment. This helps reduce the ecological footprint of your beauty routine. Many natural beauty brands are committed to cruelty-free practices, ensuring that their products are not tested on animals. This ethical approach to beauty aligns with a growing consumer demand for humane and compassionate choices.

Making your own beauty products allows you to customize them according to your specific needs and preferences. You have full control over the ingredients, ensuring purity and quality. Natural beauty brands tend to be more transparent about their ingredient lists, making it easier for consumers to know exactly what they are applying to their skin. Many natural beauty products can be made at home with simple, affordable ingredients. This can be more cost-effective than purchasing high-end commercial products.

Transitioning to a natural beauty routine doesn't have to be overwhelming. Start by replacing one product at a time, such as your moisturizer or shampoo, with a natural alternative. Pay attention to how your skin and hair respond, and enjoy the process of discovering new, nourishing products that enhance your beauty naturally.

In this ebook, you'll find 31 essential oil recipes for various cosmetic applications, each designed to harness the power of natural ingredients. From facial serums and hair growth treatments to relaxing bath soaks and soothing balms, these recipes offer a holistic approach to beauty and wellness. Embrace the benefits of natural beauty and transform your routine with these simple, effective recipes.

Welcome to a healthier, more sustainable way to care for your beauty. Let's get started!

2. ESSENTIAL OILS 101

Incorporating essential oils into your beauty routine can offer a myriad of benefits, from nourishing your skin to promoting relaxation. However, the effectiveness and safety of these oils largely depend on their quality. Choosing high-quality essential oils is crucial for reaping their full benefits, yet navigating the market can be challenging due to the lack of regulation in the industry. Many products labeled as "pure" essential oils may contain additives or be of subpar quality, which can diminish their therapeutic properties and potentially cause adverse reactions.

The essential oil industry is not strictly regulated, meaning there are no standardized guidelines for labeling or purity. As a result, some manufacturers may dilute their oils with carrier oils, synthetic fragrances, or other fillers without disclosing this on the label. This lack of transparency can make it difficult for consumers to identify truly pure essential oils. Additionally, the term "therapeutic grade" is often used as a marketing ploy, as there is no official certification for this designation.

To ensure you are purchasing high-quality essential oils, it is important to check the Latin name of the plant from which the oil is derived. This ensures you are getting the correct species and can differentiate between different varieties of the same plant. The label should state that the oil is 100% pure essential oil with no added ingredients. Be wary of terms like "fragrance oil" or "perfume oil," which indicate synthetic additives. Purchase from reputable brands known for their quality and transparency. Look for companies that provide detailed information about their sourcing, extraction methods, and testing procedures. High-quality essential oils are not cheap. If the price seems too good to be true, it probably is. Genuine essential oils require significant resources and time to produce, which is reflected in their cost. Reputable brands often perform Gas Chromatography/Mass Spectrometry (GC/MS) testing on their oils to verify purity and composition. Check if the company provides access to these test results. Essential oils should be stored in dark glass bottles to protect them from light and heat, which can degrade the oil's quality. Avoid oils sold in plastic or clear containers.

Using high-quality essential oils in your recipes is essential for achieving the desired results. Pure essential oils retain the plant's therapeutic properties, ensuring that your homemade cosmetics are effective and safe. Impure or adulterated oils may not only be less effective but can also cause skin irritation, allergic reactions, or other adverse effects. In this ebook, all recipes are designed with the assumption that you are using high-quality, pure essential oils. This ensures that the beneficial properties of the oils are fully utilized and that you can enjoy the best possible results from your homemade cosmetics.

Educating yourself about the essential oil industry and being vigilant about the products you purchase is the best way to ensure you are getting high-quality oils. Take the time to research brands, read labels carefully, and don't hesitate to reach out to manufacturers for more information about their products. By making informed choices, you can confidently incorporate essential oils into your beauty routine, knowing that you are using the best possible ingredients.

Transitioning to natural beauty products is a journey toward better health and well-being. Choosing high-quality essential oils is a crucial step in this journey. With this knowledge, you are well-equipped to navigate the essential oil market and make choices that support your goals for a healthier, more natural beauty routine. Let's continue this journey with confidence, knowing that each drop of essential oil you use is pure, potent, and beneficial for your beauty and wellness.

3. ESSENTIAL OIL RECIPES FOR THE FACE

1. Lavender, Tea Tree & Frankincense Cleanser

This Lavender, Tea Tree & Frankincense Cleanser is a gentle yet effective solution for removing impurities while nourishing your skin. The combination of jojoba oil and castile soap forms a cleansing base, while the essential oils offer soothing, antimicrobial, and rejuvenating benefits. Use this cleanser daily to maintain clean, healthy, and refreshed skin.

Ingredients:

- 1/4 cup of liquid castile soap (gentle cleanser)
- 1/4 cup of jojoba oil (moisturizing and balancing)
- 1/4 cup of distilled water (to dilute and soften)
- 5 drops of lavender essential oil (calming and soothing)
- 5 drops of tea tree essential oil (antimicrobial and clarifying)
- 5 drops of frankincense essential oil (rejuvenating and healing)
- A small funnel (optional, for easier pouring)
- A clean pump bottle or dispenser bottle

Instructions:

1. **Prepare Your Workspace**:
   - o   Ensure that your pump bottle or dispenser bottle and any mixing tools are clean and dry. Sterilizing the container by rinsing it with boiling water and letting it air dry can help prevent contamination.
2. **Combine Base Ingredients**:
   - o   In a small mixing bowl or directly in the pump bottle, combine 1/4 cup of liquid castile soap, 1/4 cup of jojoba oil, and 1/4 cup of distilled water. Stir or shake well to mix.
3. **Add Essential Oils**:
   - o   Add 5 drops of lavender essential oil, 5 drops of tea tree essential oil, and 5 drops of frankincense essential oil to the mixture. Stir thoroughly to ensure the essential oils are evenly distributed.
4. **Mix Thoroughly**:
   - o   If mixing in a bowl, stir the mixture until all ingredients are well combined. If mixing directly in the pump bottle, cap the bottle and shake well to combine all ingredients.
5. **Transfer and Store**:
   - o   If you mixed the ingredients in a bowl, use a small funnel to transfer the mixture into your pump bottle or dispenser bottle. Cap the bottle tightly.
6. **Label and Store**:
   - o   Label the bottle with the contents and date. Store the cleanser in a cool, dark place to preserve the integrity of the ingredients. The cleanser should be used within three months for the best results.

Application:

- • Wet your face with warm water.
- • Pump a small amount of the cleanser onto your fingertips or a cleansing cloth.
- • Gently massage the cleanser into your skin in circular motions, focusing on areas with makeup or impurities.
- • Rinse thoroughly with warm water and pat your face dry with a clean towel.
- • Follow up with your favorite toner and moisturizer.

Tips:

- Perform a patch test before using the cleanser to ensure you don't have any allergic reactions to the essential oils.
- Customize the blend by adjusting the essential oils to your preference, keeping the total number of drops the same.
- For added exfoliation, mix in a teaspoon of finely ground oats or almond meal.
- If you prefer a richer cleanser, add a teaspoon of vitamin E oil for additional moisturizing benefits.

This Lavender, Tea Tree & Frankincense Cleanser is a gentle and effective way of cleansing, nourishing, and refreshing your skin with essential oils and natural ingredients. Experience a clean, healthy, and rejuvenated complexion with every use.

2. Bergamot & Geranium Facial Toner

This Bergamot & Geranium Facial Toner is perfect for balancing and refreshing your skin. Bergamot essential oil helps to cleanse and balance oily skin, while geranium essential oil promotes skin health and has a calming effect. This toner can help to tighten pores, remove residual impurities, and leave your skin feeling refreshed and revitalized.

Ingredients:

- 1/2 cup of distilled water (base for the toner)
- 1/4 cup of witch hazel (natural astringent and toner)
- 1 tablespoon of aloe vera gel (soothing and hydrating)
- 5 drops of bergamot essential oil (cleansing and balancing)
- 5 drops of geranium essential oil (calming and promoting skin health)
- A small spray bottle or bottle with a lid (preferably glass)
- A small funnel (optional, for easier pouring)

Instructions:

1. **Prepare Your Workspace**:
    - Ensure that your spray bottle or container and any mixing tools are clean and dry. Sterilizing the bottle by rinsing it with boiling water and letting it air dry can help prevent contamination.
2. **Combine Liquid Ingredients**:
    - In a small bowl or directly in the spray bottle, combine 1/2 cup of distilled water, 1/4 cup of witch hazel, and 1 tablespoon of aloe vera gel. Stir or shake well to mix.
3. **Add Essential Oils**:
    - Add 5 drops of bergamot essential oil and 5 drops of geranium essential oil to the liquid mixture. Essential oils should be added carefully to ensure the correct dilution and effectiveness.

4. **Mix Thoroughly**:
   - o   If mixing in a bowl, stir the mixture thoroughly to ensure the essential oils are evenly distributed. If mixing directly in the spray bottle, cap the bottle and shake well to combine all ingredients.
5. **Transfer (if necessary) and Store**:
   - o   If you mixed the ingredients in a bowl, use a small funnel to transfer the mixture into your spray bottle or container. Cap the bottle tightly.
6. **Label and Store**:
   - o   Label the bottle with the contents and date. Store the facial toner in a cool, dark place to preserve the integrity of the ingredients. The toner should be used within three months for the best results.

Application:

- Cleanse your face thoroughly before applying the toner.
- Apply the toner to a cotton pad and gently sweep it across your face and neck, avoiding the eye area.
- Alternatively, if using a spray bottle, close your eyes and mist the toner evenly over your face and neck.
- Allow the toner to absorb into your skin before applying moisturizer or other skincare products.
- Use the toner morning and night as part of your skincare routine.

Tips:

- Perform a patch test before using the facial toner to ensure you don't have any allergic reactions to the essential oils.
- Shake the bottle well before each use to ensure the essential oils are evenly distributed.
- Customize the scent by adjusting the essential oils to your preference, keeping the total number of drops the same.
- If you have sensitive skin, consider reducing the amount of witch hazel or using an alcohol-free version.

This Bergamot & Geranium Facial Toner will leave you with a clean, refreshed feeling and healthy, glowing.

---

3. Lavender & Frankincense Tinted Moisturizer

This Lavender & Frankincense Tinted Moisturizer is designed to hydrate your skin while providing a subtle, natural tint. Lavender essential oil offers soothing and calming properties, while frankincense essential oil helps to rejuvenate and tone the skin. Combined with a nourishing base and natural pigments, this tinted moisturizer will leave your skin looking healthy and radiant.

Ingredients:

- 2 tablespoons of your favorite natural moisturizer (such as aloe vera gel, shea butter, or a lightweight lotion)
- 1 teaspoon of non-nano zinc oxide (for sun protection)
- 1 teaspoon of cocoa powder (for tint)
- 1-2 drops of lavender essential oil (for soothing and calming the skin)
- 1-2 drops of frankincense essential oil (for anti-aging and skin rejuvenation)
- 1-2 drops of tea tree essential oil (optional, for acne-prone skin)

Instructions:

1. **Prepare Your Base:**
   - In a small bowl, add 2 tablespoons of your natural moisturizer. Aloe vera gel or a lightweight, non-greasy lotion works well for a tinted moisturizer.
2. **Add Sun Protection:**
   - Mix in 1 teaspoon of non-nano zinc oxide. This ingredient provides a physical barrier against UV rays, offering sun protection without the need for chemical sunscreens. Be careful not to inhale the powder during this step.
3. **Create the Tint:**

- o Gradually add 1 teaspoon of cocoa powder to the mixture, blending thoroughly. Adjust the amount based on your desired shade. Start with a small amount and add more as needed until you reach your preferred level of tint.

4. **Incorporate Essential Oils**:
   - o Add 1-2 drops of lavender essential oil to the mixture for its soothing and calming properties. Lavender is gentle on the skin and helps reduce redness and irritation.
   - o Add 1-2 drops of frankincense essential oil for its anti-aging and skin rejuvenating benefits. Frankincense promotes cell regeneration and improves skin elasticity.
   - o If you have acne-prone skin, you can also add 1-2 drops of tea tree essential oil. Tea tree oil has antibacterial properties that help combat acne and prevent breakouts.

5. **Mix and Store**:
   - o Thoroughly mix all the ingredients until you achieve a smooth, even consistency. Ensure that the cocoa powder is well blended to avoid streaks in the moisturizer.
   - o Transfer the tinted moisturizer into a clean, airtight container. A small glass jar or a pump bottle works well for easy application and storage.

Application:

- Apply the tinted moisturizer to your face as you would with any moisturizer. Start with a small amount and blend evenly over your skin. The tint should provide light coverage, evening out your skin tone while keeping your skin hydrated and protected.

Tips:

- Customize the shade by adjusting the amount of cocoa powder to match your skin tone.
- If you prefer a dewy finish, add a few drops of jojoba oil or argan oil to the mixture.
- For a matte finish, incorporate a small amount of arrowroot powder or cornstarch to the recipe.

This Lavender & Frankincense Tinted Moisturizer is a luxurious enhancement to your skincare routine, offering hydration, a natural tint, and the soothing benefits of premium essential oils and natural ingredients. Revel in the healthy, radiant glow it imparts.

13

4. Frankincense & Myrrh Anti-Aging Night Cream

This luxurious Frankincense & Myrrh Anti-Aging Night Cream combines the powerful anti-aging properties of essential oils with nourishing carrier oils and butters to create a rich, hydrating cream that promotes youthful, radiant skin. Frankincense essential oil helps reduce the appearance of fine lines and wrinkles, while myrrh essential oil rejuvenates and revitalizes the skin.

Ingredients:

- 1/4 cup of shea butter (deeply moisturizing and rich in vitamins A and E)
- 2 tablespoons of coconut oil (hydrates and protects the skin)
- 1 tablespoon of jojoba oil (mimics the skin's natural oils)
- 1 tablespoon of rosehip oil (rich in essential fatty acids and antioxidants)
- 10 drops of frankincense essential oil
- 10 drops of myrrh essential oil
- 1 teaspoon of vitamin E oil (optional, for added antioxidant benefits)
- A double boiler or heat-safe bowl and saucepan
- A hand mixer or whisk
- A small glass jar or container with a lid

Instructions:

1. **Prepare Your Workspace**:
   - Ensure that your glass jar or container and any mixing tools are clean and dry. Sterilizing the jar by rinsing it with boiling water and letting it air dry can help prevent contamination.
2. **Melt the Shea Butter and Coconut Oil**:
   - In a double boiler or a heat-safe bowl set over a saucepan of simmering water, melt 1/4 cup of shea butter and 2 tablespoons of coconut oil. Stir occasionally until fully melted and combined.

3. **Add the Carrier Oils**:
   o Remove the melted shea butter and coconut oil from heat. Add 1 tablespoon of jojoba oil and 1 tablespoon of rosehip oil to the mixture. Stir well to combine.
4. **Incorporate Essential Oils**:
   o Allow the mixture to cool slightly but not solidify. Add 10 drops of frankincense essential oil and 10 drops of myrrh essential oil to the mixture. If using, add 1 teaspoon of vitamin E oil for its additional antioxidant benefits.
5. **Mix and Whip**:
   o Using a hand mixer or whisk, blend the mixture until it becomes creamy and smooth. This may take a few minutes and will help to create a light, whipped texture for the cream.
6. **Transfer and Store**:
   o Carefully transfer the whipped cream into your glass jar or container using a spatula. Ensure the jar is filled and sealed tightly with a lid.
7. **Label and Store**:
   o Label the jar with the contents and date. Store the cream in a cool, dark place to preserve the integrity of the oils and butters. The cream should be used within six months for the best results.

Application:

- Apply a small amount of the cream to your face and neck after cleansing and toning, preferably in the evening before bedtime.
- Gently massage the cream into your skin using upward, circular motions.
- Allow the cream to absorb fully before applying any other products or makeup.

Tips:

- For an added cooling effect, store the cream in the refrigerator.
- Perform a patch test before using the cream on your face to ensure you don't have any allergic reactions to the essential oils.
- Use consistently for best results, as the anti-aging effects will improve over time.

This Frankincense & Myrrh Anti-Aging Night Cream is a luxurious addition to your skincare routine, providing your skin with the powerful benefits of high-quality essential oils and nourishing butters. Enjoy the rejuvenating experience and the radiant, youthful skin that follows.

5. Rose & Chamomile Eye Cream

This Rose & Chamomile Eye Cream is designed to soothe and hydrate the delicate skin around your eyes. Rose essential oil has anti-inflammatory and moisturizing properties, while chamomile essential oil is known for its calming and soothing effects. Combined with nourishing shea butter and oils, this eye cream will help reduce puffiness and fine lines, leaving your eye area looking refreshed and rejuvenated.

Ingredients:

- 2 tablespoons of shea butter (deeply moisturizing and rich in vitamins A and E)
- 1 tablespoon of coconut oil (hydrates and protects the skin)
- 1 tablespoon of sweet almond oil (lightweight and easily absorbed)
- 10 drops of rose essential oil (anti-inflammatory and moisturizing)
- 5 drops of chamomile essential oil (calming and soothing)
- 1 teaspoon of vitamin E oil (optional, for added skin benefits)
- A double boiler or heat-safe bowl and saucepan
- A hand mixer or whisk
- A clean glass jar or container with a lid

Instructions:

1. **Prepare Your Workspace:**
   - Ensure that your glass jar or container and any mixing tools are clean and dry. Sterilizing the jar by rinsing it with boiling water and letting it air dry can help prevent contamination.
2. **Melt the Shea Butter and Coconut Oil:**
   - In a double boiler or a heat-safe bowl set over a saucepan of simmering water, melt 2 tablespoons of shea butter and 1

tablespoon of coconut oil. Stir occasionally until fully melted and combined.

3. **Add Sweet Almond Oil**:
   o Remove the melted shea butter and coconut oil from heat. Add 1 tablespoon of sweet almond oil to the mixture and stir well to combine.

4. **Cool Slightly and Add Essential Oils**:
   o Allow the mixture to cool slightly but not solidify. Add 10 drops of rose essential oil and 5 drops of chamomile essential oil. If using, add 1 teaspoon of vitamin E oil. Stir well to ensure the essential oils and vitamin E oil are evenly distributed.

5. **Mix and Whip**:
   o Using a hand mixer or whisk, blend the mixture until it becomes creamy and smooth. This may take a few minutes and will help to create a light, whipped texture for the eye cream.

6. **Transfer and Store**:
   o Carefully transfer the whipped eye cream into your glass jar or container using a spatula. Ensure the jar is filled and sealed tightly with a lid.

7. **Label and Store**:
   o Label the jar with the contents and date. Store the eye cream in a cool, dark place to preserve the integrity of the oils and butters. The eye cream should be used within six months for the best results.

Application:

- Apply a small amount of the eye cream to the skin around your eyes using your ring finger, which applies the least pressure.
- Gently pat the cream into your skin, focusing on areas with puffiness and fine lines.
- Use the eye cream daily, preferably in the evening before bed, for best results.

Tips:

- Perform a patch test before using the eye cream to ensure you don't have any allergic reactions to the essential oils.

- For an added cooling effect, store the eye cream in the refrigerator.
- Customize the scent by adjusting the essential oils to your preference, keeping the total number of drops the same.
- If you prefer a firmer eye cream, increase the amount of shea butter slightly.

This Rose & Chamomile Eye Cream adds a touch of luxury to your skincare routine, offering your eye area the soothing and moisturizing benefits of premium essential oils and natural ingredients. Revel in the refreshed, youthful appearance it brings.

6. Lavender & Chamomile Facial Serum

This Lavender & Chamomile Facial Serum is designed to soothe and hydrate your skin, making it perfect for all skin types, especially sensitive and irritated skin. Lavender essential oil helps to calm and heal the skin, while chamomile essential oil reduces redness and inflammation. This lightweight serum absorbs quickly, leaving your skin feeling soft and refreshed.

Ingredients:

- 1 tablespoon of jojoba oil (carrier oil)
- 1 tablespoon of argan oil (carrier oil)
- 10 drops of lavender essential oil
- 10 drops of chamomile essential oil
- 1 teaspoon of vitamin E oil (optional, for added skin benefits)
- A small dropper bottle (preferably amber or cobalt blue to protect the oils from light)

Instructions:

1. **Prepare Your Workspace:**
   - Ensure that your dropper bottle and any mixing tools are clean and dry. Sterilizing the bottle by rinsing it with boiling water and letting it air dry can help prevent contamination.
2. **Measure and Combine Carrier Oils:**
   - In a small bowl or directly in the dropper bottle, combine 1 tablespoon of jojoba oil and 1 tablespoon of argan oil. These carrier oils are chosen for their lightweight, non-comedogenic properties and their ability to nourish and hydrate the skin without clogging pores.
3. **Add Essential Oils:**

- o   Add 10 drops of lavender essential oil to the carrier oils. Lavender oil is known for its calming and healing properties, making it ideal for soothing irritated or sensitive skin.
  - o   Add 10 drops of chamomile essential oil. Chamomile oil helps reduce redness and inflammation, promoting a more even complexion.

4. **Optional: Add Vitamin E Oil**:
   - o   Add 1 teaspoon of vitamin E oil if desired. Vitamin E is an antioxidant that helps protect the skin from free radical damage and enhances the serum's moisturizing properties.

5. **Mix and Transfer**:
   - o   Mix the oils thoroughly to ensure that the essential oils are evenly distributed throughout the carrier oils.
   - o   Carefully transfer the mixture into your dropper bottle using a small funnel if necessary.

6. **Label and Store**:
   - o   Label the dropper bottle with the contents and date. Store the serum in a cool, dark place to preserve the integrity of the oils. The serum should be used within six months for the best results.

Application:

- Apply a few drops of the serum to clean, dry skin, preferably in the evening before bedtime.
- Gently massage the serum into your face and neck using upward, circular motions.
- Allow the serum to absorb fully before applying any other products or makeup.

Tips:

- For an added cooling effect, store the serum in the refrigerator.
- Perform a patch test before using the serum on your face to ensure you don't have any allergic reactions to the essential oils.
- Use consistently for best results, as the calming and hydrating effects will improve over time.

This Lavender & Chamomile Facial Serum, provides your skin with the calming and healing benefits of high-quality essential oils and nourishing carrier oils. Enjoy the soothing experience and the radiant, healthy skin that follows.

7. Geranium & Ylang Ylang Facial Oil

This Geranium & Ylang Ylang Facial Oil is designed to balance, hydrate, and rejuvenate your skin. Geranium essential oil helps regulate sebum production and improves skin elasticity, while ylang ylang essential oil soothes and enhances skin health. Combined with nourishing carrier oils, this facial oil will leave your skin feeling soft, smooth, and radiant.

Ingredients:

- 2 tablespoons of jojoba oil (balances sebum production and is easily absorbed)
- 1 tablespoon of rosehip oil (rich in vitamins and antioxidants)
- 1 tablespoon of argan oil (moisturizes and improves skin elasticity)
- 10 drops of geranium essential oil (regulates sebum and improves skin elasticity)
- 5 drops of ylang ylang essential oil (soothes and enhances skin health)
- A small glass dropper bottle
- A small funnel (optional, for easier pouring)

Instructions:

1. **Prepare Your Workspace:**
   - Ensure that your dropper bottle and any mixing tools are clean and dry. Sterilizing the bottle by rinsing it with boiling water and letting it air dry can help prevent contamination.
2. **Combine Carrier Oils:**
   - In a small bowl or directly in the dropper bottle, combine 2 tablespoons of jojoba oil, 1 tablespoon of rosehip oil, and 1 tablespoon of argan oil. Stir or shake well to mix.
3. **Add Essential Oils:**

o   Add 10 drops of geranium essential oil and 5 drops of ylang ylang essential oil to the mixture. Essential oils should be added carefully to ensure the correct dilution and effectiveness.

4. **Mix Thoroughly**:

o   If mixing in a bowl, stir the mixture thoroughly to ensure the essential oils are evenly distributed. If mixing directly in the dropper bottle, cap the bottle and shake well to combine all ingredients.

5. **Transfer (if necessary) and Store**:

o   If you mixed the ingredients in a bowl, use a small funnel to transfer the mixture into your dropper bottle. Cap the bottle tightly.

6. **Label and Store**:

o   Label the dropper bottle with the contents and date. Store the facial oil in a cool, dark place to preserve the integrity of the oils. The facial oil should be used within six months for the best results.

Application:

- After cleansing and toning your face, apply a few drops of the facial oil to your fingertips.
- Gently massage the oil into your skin using upward, circular motions, focusing on areas that need extra hydration and care.
- Use the facial oil daily, preferably in the evening, for best results.

Tips:

- Perform a patch test before using the facial oil to ensure you don't have any allergic reactions to the essential oils.
- Customize the scent by adjusting the essential oils to your preference, keeping the total number of drops the same.
- For an added cooling effect, store the facial oil in the refrigerator.
- If you prefer a lighter oil, reduce the amount of rosehip oil slightly and increase the amount of jojoba or argan oil.

This Geranium & Ylang Ylang Facial Oil is a luxurious addition to your skincare routine, offering your skin balance, hydration, and rejuvenation. Experience a soft, smooth, and radiant complexion with every use.

8. Rose & Sandalwood Face Mist

This Rose & Sandalwood Face Mist is designed to hydrate and refresh your skin while providing a calming and luxurious scent. Rose essential oil helps to soothe and balance the skin, while sandalwood essential oil offers anti-inflammatory and moisturizing properties. This mist is perfect for a quick pick-me-up throughout the day or as a hydrating toner in your skincare routine.

Ingredients:

- 1/2 cup of distilled water (base for the face mist)
- 1/4 cup of rose water (soothing and hydrating)
- 1 tablespoon of witch hazel (natural astringent and toner)
- 5 drops of rose essential oil (soothing and balancing)
- 5 drops of sandalwood essential oil (anti-inflammatory and moisturizing)
- A small spray bottle (preferably glass)
- A small funnel (optional, for easier pouring)

Instructions:

1. **Prepare Your Workspace**:
   - Ensure that your spray bottle and any mixing tools are clean and dry. Sterilizing the bottle by rinsing it with boiling water and letting it air dry can help prevent contamination.
2. **Combine Liquid Ingredients**:
   - In a small bowl or directly in the spray bottle, combine 1/2 cup of distilled water, 1/4 cup of rose water, and 1 tablespoon of witch hazel. Stir or shake well to mix.
3. **Add Essential Oils**:
   - Add 5 drops of rose essential oil and 5 drops of sandalwood essential oil to the liquid mixture. Essential oils should be added carefully to ensure the correct dilution and effectiveness.

4. **Mix Thoroughly**:
   - o   If mixing in a bowl, stir the mixture thoroughly to ensure the essential oils are evenly distributed. If mixing directly in the spray bottle, cap the bottle and shake well to combine all ingredients.
5. **Transfer (if necessary) and Store**:
   - o   If you mixed the ingredients in a bowl, use a small funnel to transfer the mixture into your spray bottle. Cap the bottle tightly.
6. **Label and Store**:
   - o   Label the spray bottle with the contents and date. Store the face mist in a cool, dark place to preserve the integrity of the ingredients. The mist should be used within three months for the best results.

Application:

- Close your eyes and spray the mist evenly across your face from about 12 inches away.
- Use the face mist as a toner after cleansing your face or as a refreshing spray throughout the day.
- Allow the mist to absorb into your skin naturally, or gently pat it in with your fingertips.

Tips:

- Perform a patch test before using the face mist to ensure you don't have any allergic reactions to the essential oils.
- Shake the bottle well before each use to ensure the essential oils are evenly distributed.
- For an added cooling effect, store the face mist in the refrigerator.
- Customize the scent by adjusting the essential oils to your preference, keeping the total number of drops the same.

This Rose & Sandalwood Face Mist is a delightful addition to your skincare routine, providing your skin with the hydrating and soothing benefits of high-quality essential oils and natural ingredients. Enjoy the refreshing, luxurious feel and the radiant, hydrated skin that follows.

9. This Lavendar & Geranium Blusher

This Lavender & Geranium Blusher offers a natural, radiant glow with the soothing and balancing properties of essential oils. The combination of beetroot powder and arrowroot powder provides a beautiful pink hue, while the essential oils add a subtle, pleasant scent and skin benefits.

Ingredients:

- 1 tablespoon of arrowroot powder (for a smooth texture)
- 1 teaspoon of beetroot powder (for natural color)
- 1/2 teaspoon of kaolin clay (for a matte finish)
- 2 drops of lavender essential oil (soothing and calming)
- 2 drops of geranium essential oil (balancing and nourishing)
- A small mixing bowl
- A clean container with a lid

Instructions:

1. **Prepare Your Workspace:**
   o Ensure that your container and any mixing tools are clean and dry. Sterilizing the container by rinsing it with boiling water and letting it air dry can help prevent contamination.
2. **Combine Dry Ingredients:**
   o In a small mixing bowl, combine 1 tablespoon of arrowroot powder, 1 teaspoon of beetroot powder, and 1/2 teaspoon of kaolin clay. Mix well to ensure the powders are evenly distributed.
3. **Add Essential Oils:**
   o Add 2 drops of lavender essential oil and 2 drops of geranium essential oil to the mixture. Stir thoroughly to ensure the essential oils are evenly dispersed.
4. **Mix Thoroughly:**

- o   Continue to stir the mixture until all ingredients are well combined and the texture is consistent.

5. **Transfer and Store**:
   - o   Carefully transfer the blusher into your clean container using a spatula or spoon. Ensure the container is filled and sealed tightly with a lid.

6. **Label and Store**:
   - o   Label the container with the contents and date. Store the blusher in a cool, dark place to preserve the integrity of the ingredients. The blusher should be used within six months for the best results.

Application:

- Using a clean makeup brush, apply a small amount of the blusher to the apples of your cheeks.
- Blend well using circular motions to achieve a natural, radiant glow.
- Adjust the intensity of the color by applying more or less blusher as desired.

Tips:

- Perform a patch test before using the blusher to ensure you don't have any allergic reactions to the essential oils.
- Customize the color by adjusting the amount of beetroot powder or adding a small amount of cocoa powder for a deeper hue.
- For a shimmery finish, add a pinch of mica powder to the mixture.
- If you prefer a cream blusher, add a small amount of jojoba oil and mix well to achieve the desired consistency.

This Lavender & Geranium Blusher is a beautiful and healthy addition to your makeup routine, providing your cheeks with a natural, radiant glow. Enjoy the vibrant, fresh look.

10. Lavender, Rosemary & Cedarwood Eyelash Growth Serum

This Lavender, Rosemary & Cedarwood Eyelash Growth Serum is formulated to nourish and strengthen your eyelashes, promoting natural growth and enhancing their appearance. Castor oil and coconut oil serve as the nourishing base, while the essential oils provide additional benefits to support healthy lash growth.

Ingredients:

- 2 tablespoons of castor oil (promotes hair growth and strengthens lashes)
- 1 tablespoon of coconut oil (moisturizes and nourishes)
- 3 drops of lavender essential oil (conditions and promotes healthy hair growth)
- 3 drops of rosemary essential oil (stimulates hair follicles)
- 3 drops of cedarwood essential oil (supports hair growth and strengthens)
- A clean mascara tube or small dropper bottle
- A small funnel (optional, for easier pouring)

Instructions:

1. **Prepare Your Workspace:**
   - Ensure that your mascara tube or dropper bottle and any mixing tools are clean and dry. Sterilizing the container by rinsing it with boiling water and letting it air dry can help prevent contamination.
2. **Combine Carrier Oils:**
   - In a small mixing bowl, combine 2 tablespoons of castor oil and 1 tablespoon of coconut oil. Stir well to mix.
3. **Add Essential Oils:**

     o   Add 3 drops of lavender essential oil, 3 drops of rosemary essential oil, and 3 drops of cedarwood essential oil to the mixture. Stir thoroughly to ensure the essential oils are evenly distributed.

4. **Mix Thoroughly**:
    - Continue to stir the mixture until all ingredients are well combined and the texture is consistent.

5. **Transfer and Store**:
    - Carefully transfer the eyelash growth serum into your clean mascara tube or dropper bottle using a funnel if needed. Ensure the container is filled and sealed tightly with a lid.

6. **Label and Store**:
    - Label the container with the contents and date. Store the serum in a cool, dark place to preserve the integrity of the oils. The serum should be used within six months for the best results.

Application:

- Ensure your eyelashes are clean and free of makeup.
- Using the mascara wand or a clean fingertip, apply a small amount of the serum to the base of your upper and lower lashes.
- Be careful to avoid getting the serum in your eyes.
- Use the serum nightly before bed for the best results.

Tips:

- Perform a patch test before using the serum to ensure you don't have any allergic reactions to the essential oils.
- For best results, use consistently every night.
- If you prefer a lighter serum, increase the amount of coconut oil slightly.
- Ensure to always handle the applicator with clean hands to avoid contamination.

This Lavender, Rosemary & Cedarwood Eyelash Growth Serum is a natural and effective way to nourish and strengthen your lashes, promoting healthy growth and enhancing their appearance. Enjoy the fuller, longer lashes it helps to achieve.

11. Peppermint & Lemon Lip Scrub

This Peppermint & Lemon Lip Scrub is designed to exfoliate and rejuvenate your lips, leaving them smooth and refreshed. Peppermint essential oil provides a cooling and invigorating sensation, while lemon essential oil brightens and revitalizes. Combined with sugar for gentle exfoliation and coconut oil for hydration, this lip scrub will keep your lips soft and supple.

Ingredients:

- 2 tablespoons of granulated sugar (exfoliating agent)
- 1 tablespoon of coconut oil (moisturizing and nourishing)
- 5 drops of peppermint essential oil (cooling and invigorating)
- 5 drops of lemon essential oil (brightening and revitalizing)
- 1/2 teaspoon of honey (optional, for added moisture and antibacterial properties)
- A small mixing bowl
- A clean glass jar or container with a lid

Instructions:

1. **Prepare Your Workspace:**
   - Ensure that your glass jar or container and any mixing tools are clean and dry. Sterilizing the jar by rinsing it with boiling water and letting it air dry can help prevent contamination.
2. **Combine Sugar and Coconut Oil:**
   - In a small mixing bowl, combine 2 tablespoons of granulated sugar and 1 tablespoon of coconut oil. Mix thoroughly until the sugar is evenly coated with the oil. The coconut oil should be in a semi-solid state; if it's too solid, you can soften it slightly by warming it in a microwave or over a double boiler.
3. **Add Essential Oils:**

- o Add 5 drops of peppermint essential oil to the sugar and coconut oil mixture. Peppermint oil provides a refreshing, cooling sensation.
  - o Add 5 drops of lemon essential oil. Lemon oil brightens and revitalizes the lips, giving the scrub a refreshing citrus scent.

4. **Optional: Add Honey**:
   - o For added moisture and antibacterial properties, mix in 1/2 teaspoon of honey. The honey also helps to bind the ingredients together.

5. **Mix Thoroughly**:
   - o Stir the mixture until all the ingredients are well combined and the essential oils are evenly distributed throughout the sugar and coconut oil.

6. **Transfer and Store**:
   - o Carefully transfer the lip scrub into your glass jar or container using a spatula. Ensure the jar is filled and sealed tightly with a lid.

7. **Label and Store**:
   - o Label the jar with the contents and date. Store the lip scrub in a cool, dark place to preserve the integrity of the ingredients. The scrub should be used within three months for the best results.

Application:

- Apply a small amount of the lip scrub to clean, dry lips.
- Gently massage the scrub into your lips using circular motions to exfoliate and remove dead skin cells.
- Rinse thoroughly with warm water and pat dry.
- Follow up with a hydrating lip balm for best results.
- Use the lip scrub 1-2 times a week for smooth, soft lips.

Tips:

- Perform a patch test before using the lip scrub to ensure you don't have any allergic reactions to the essential oils.
- If you prefer a finer scrub, you can use a smaller granulated sugar.
- Customize the scent by adjusting the essential oils to your preference, keeping the total number of drops the same.

- Store the lip scrub in an airtight container to keep it fresh and prevent the essential oils from evaporating.

This Peppermint & Lemon Lip Scrub is a delightful addition to your lip care routine, providing your lips with the exfoliating and refreshing benefits of high-quality essential oils and natural ingredients to create smooth and soft lips.

12. Patchouli & Orange Lip Balm

This Patchouli & Orange Lip Balm combines the earthy, grounding scent of patchouli with the uplifting, citrusy aroma of orange. It provides deep hydration and protection for your lips, leaving them soft and smooth. The natural ingredients in this lip balm are gentle and nourishing, perfect for everyday use.

Ingredients:

- 2 tablespoons of beeswax pellets (provides structure and protection)
- 2 tablespoons of shea butter (deeply moisturizing and rich in vitamins)
- 2 tablespoons of coconut oil (hydrates and protects the lips)
- 10 drops of patchouli essential oil (grounding and moisturizing)
- 10 drops of orange essential oil (uplifting and brightening)
- A double boiler or heat-safe bowl and saucepan
- Lip balm containers or tubes

Instructions:

1. **Prepare Your Workspace**:
   - Ensure that your lip balm containers or tubes and any mixing tools are clean and dry. Sterilizing the containers by rinsing them with boiling water and letting them air dry can help prevent contamination.
2. **Melt the Beeswax, Shea Butter, and Coconut Oil**:
   - In a double boiler or a heat-safe bowl set over a saucepan of simmering water, melt 2 tablespoons of beeswax pellets, 2 tablespoons of shea butter, and 2 tablespoons of coconut oil. Stir occasionally until fully melted and combined.
3. **Remove from Heat and Add Essential Oils**:
   - Once the mixture is melted and well combined, remove it from heat. Allow it to cool slightly but not solidify. Add 10 drops of

patchouli essential oil and 10 drops of orange essential oil to the mixture. Stir well to ensure the essential oils are evenly distributed.

4. **Pour into Containers**:
    o   Carefully pour the mixture into your lip balm containers or tubes using a small funnel or pipette if necessary. Fill each container to the top, as the mixture will shrink slightly as it cools.
5. **Cool and Solidify**:
    o   Allow the lip balm to cool and solidify completely at room temperature. This may take a few hours. Once solidified, cap the containers or tubes tightly.
6. **Label and Store**:
    o   Label the containers with the contents and date. Store the lip balm in a cool, dark place to preserve the integrity of the oils and butters. The lip balm should be used within six months for the best results.

Tips:

- Perform a patch test before using the lip balm to ensure you don't have any allergic reactions to the essential oils.
- If you prefer a softer lip balm, reduce the amount of beeswax slightly.
- Customize the scent by adjusting the essential oils to your preference, keeping the total number of drops the same.
- Consider making a larger batch and giving the lip balms as gifts to friends and family.

This Patchouli & Orange Lip Balm is a wonderful addition to your natural beauty routine, providing your lips with the nourishing and protective benefits of high-quality essential oils and moisturizing butters. Enjoy the unique, delightful scent and wonderfully hydrated and soft lips.

13. Cedarwood & Bergamot Makeup Setting Spray

This Cedarwood & Bergamot Makeup Setting Spray helps to set your makeup while providing a refreshing and uplifting scent. Cedarwood essential oil has calming and balancing properties, while bergamot essential oil provides a fresh, citrusy aroma. This spray can help to keep your makeup in place and leave your skin feeling hydrated and revitalized.

Ingredients:

- 1/2 cup of distilled water (base for the spray)
- 1/4 cup of witch hazel (natural astringent and helps set makeup)
- 1 tablespoon of aloe vera gel (soothing and hydrating)
- 5 drops of cedarwood essential oil (calming and balancing)
- 5 drops of bergamot essential oil (refreshing and uplifting)
- A small spray bottle (preferably glass)
- A small funnel (optional, for easier pouring)

Instructions:

1. **Prepare Your Workspace**:
   - Ensure that your spray bottle and any mixing tools are clean and dry. Sterilizing the bottle by rinsing it with boiling water and letting it air dry can help prevent contamination.
2. **Combine Liquid Ingredients**:
   - In a small bowl or directly in the spray bottle, combine 1/2 cup of distilled water, 1/4 cup of witch hazel, and 1 tablespoon of aloe vera gel. Stir or shake well to mix.
3. **Add Essential Oils**:
   - Add 5 drops of cedarwood essential oil and 5 drops of bergamot essential oil to the liquid mixture. Essential oils should be added carefully to ensure the correct dilution and effectiveness.

4. **Mix Thoroughly**:
    o   If mixing in a bowl, stir the mixture thoroughly to ensure the essential oils are evenly distributed. If mixing directly in the spray bottle, cap the bottle and shake well to combine all ingredients.
5. **Transfer (if necessary) and Store**:
    o   If you mixed the ingredients in a bowl, use a small funnel to transfer the mixture into your spray bottle. Cap the bottle tightly.
6. **Label and Store**:
    o   Label the spray bottle with the contents and date. Store the setting spray in a cool, dark place to preserve the integrity of the ingredients. The spray should be used within three months for the best results.

Application:

- After applying your makeup, hold the bottle about 12 inches away from your face.
- Close your eyes and mist the setting spray evenly over your face, using 3-4 sprays to cover the entire area.
- Allow the spray to dry naturally, or gently pat it into your skin with clean hands.
- Use the setting spray as needed throughout the day to refresh your makeup and hydrate your skin.

Tips:

- Perform a patch test before using the setting spray to ensure you don't have any allergic reactions to the essential oils.
- Shake the bottle well before each use to ensure the essential oils are evenly distributed.
- Customize the scent by adjusting the essential oils to your preference, keeping the total number of drops the same.
- For an added cooling effect, store the setting spray in the refrigerator.

This Cedarwood & Bergamot Makeup Setting Spray is a fantastic addition to your makeup bag, helping to set your makeup and keep your skin feeling fresh and hydrated.

14. Tea Tree & Lemon Acne Spot Treatment

This Tea Tree & Lemon Acne Spot Treatment is designed to target and reduce acne breakouts effectively. Tea tree essential oil has powerful antibacterial properties, while lemon essential oil helps to brighten and clarify the skin. This simple yet potent recipe can be used to spot-treat acne-prone areas, reducing inflammation and promoting clearer skin.

Ingredients:

- 2 tablespoons of aloe vera gel (soothing and healing)
- 5 drops of tea tree essential oil (antibacterial and anti-inflammatory)
- 5 drops of lemon essential oil (brightening and clarifying)
- A small glass bottle with a dropper or rollerball applicator

Instructions:

1. **Prepare Your Workspace**:
   - Ensure that your glass bottle and any mixing tools are clean and dry. Sterilizing the bottle by rinsing it with boiling water and letting it air dry can help prevent contamination.
2. **Combine the Base Ingredient**:
   - In a small bowl, add 2 tablespoons of aloe vera gel. Aloe vera gel acts as a soothing base that helps to deliver the essential oils to the skin effectively.
3. **Add Essential Oils**:
   - Add 5 drops of tea tree essential oil to the aloe vera gel. Tea tree oil is known for its antibacterial and anti-inflammatory properties, making it ideal for treating acne.
   - Add 5 drops of lemon essential oil. Lemon oil helps to brighten the skin and reduce the appearance of acne scars, but it should be used sparingly due to its potential for photosensitivity.

4. **Mix Thoroughly**:
   - Mix the aloe vera gel and essential oils thoroughly until the mixture is well combined. Ensure the essential oils are evenly distributed throughout the gel.
5. **Transfer and Store**:
   - Carefully transfer the mixture into your glass bottle using a small funnel if necessary. A dropper or rollerball applicator bottle is ideal for easy application.
6. **Label and Store**:
   - Label the bottle with the contents and date. Store the treatment in a cool, dark place to preserve the integrity of the oils. The treatment should be used within six months for the best results.

Application:

- Cleanse your face thoroughly before application.
- Apply a small amount of the spot treatment directly to acne-prone areas using the dropper or rollerball applicator.
- Gently massage the treatment into the skin and allow it to absorb.
- Use the spot treatment once or twice daily as needed. If applying during the day, ensure you follow up with sunscreen, as lemon oil can increase photosensitivity.

Tips:

- Perform a patch test before using the spot treatment to ensure you don't have any allergic reactions to the essential oils.
- Avoid sun exposure immediately after applying the treatment due to the lemon oil's photosensitivity properties. It's best to use the treatment in the evening if possible.
- Consistency is key; regular use of the spot treatment will yield the best results over time.

The Tea Tree & Lemon Acne Spot Treatment ingredients can effectively target and reduce acne breakouts, promoting clearer, healthier skin. Enjoy the benefits of this simple yet potent remedy as part of your skincare routine.

15. Lavender & Chamomile Makeup Remover

This Lavender & Chamomile Makeup Remover is designed to gently and effectively remove makeup while nourishing your skin. The combination of jojoba oil and sweet almond oil serves as the base, dissolving makeup and impurities, while lavender and chamomile essential oils provide soothing and calming benefits.

Ingredients:

- 1/4 cup of jojoba oil (dissolves makeup and balances skin)
- 1/4 cup of sweet almond oil (nourishes and moisturizes)
- 5 drops of lavender essential oil (calming and soothing)
- 5 drops of chamomile essential oil (anti-inflammatory and calming)
- A small funnel (optional, for easier pouring)
- A clean glass bottle or dispenser bottle

Instructions:

1. **Prepare Your Workspace**:
   - Ensure that your glass bottle or dispenser bottle and any mixing tools are clean and dry. Sterilizing the container by rinsing it with boiling water and letting it air dry can help prevent contamination.
2. **Combine Base Oils**:
   - In a small mixing bowl or directly in the glass bottle, combine 1/4 cup of jojoba oil and 1/4 cup of sweet almond oil. Stir or shake well to mix.
3. **Add Essential Oils**:
   - Add 5 drops of lavender essential oil and 5 drops of chamomile essential oil to the mixture. Stir thoroughly to ensure the essential oils are evenly distributed.
4. **Mix Thoroughly**:

o   If mixing in a bowl, stir the mixture until all ingredients are well combined. If mixing directly in the glass bottle, cap the bottle and shake well to combine all ingredients.

5. **Transfer and Store**:

   o   If you mixed the ingredients in a bowl, use a small funnel to transfer the mixture into your glass bottle or dispenser bottle. Cap the bottle tightly.

6. **Label and Store**:

   o   Label the bottle with the contents and date. Store the makeup remover in a cool, dark place to preserve the integrity of the ingredients. The makeup remover should be used within six months for the best results.

Application:

- Shake the bottle well before each use.
- Apply a small amount of the makeup remover to a cotton pad or a clean cloth.
- Gently wipe over your face, focusing on areas with makeup, until all makeup is removed.
- Rinse your face with warm water and pat dry.
- Follow up with your favorite cleanser and moisturizer.

Tips:

- Perform a patch test before using the makeup remover to ensure you don't have any allergic reactions to the essential oils.
- Customize the blend by adjusting the essential oils to your preference, keeping the total number of drops the same.
- If you have oily skin, consider adding a teaspoon of witch hazel for its astringent properties.
- For a refreshing boost, add a few drops of rose water to the mixture.

This Lavender & Chamomile Makeup Remover is a gentle yet powerful addition to your skincare routine, delivering the cleansing and nourishing benefits of premium essential oils and natural ingredients to your skin

4. ESSENTIAL OIL RECIPES FOR THE HAIR

16. Rosemary & Peppermint Hair Growth Serum

This Rosemary & Peppermint Hair Growth Serum is formulated to stimulate hair follicles, promote healthy hair growth, and improve scalp health. Rosemary essential oil enhances hair thickness and growth, while peppermint essential oil increases blood circulation to the scalp, promoting healthier hair follicles.

Ingredients:

- 2 tablespoons of castor oil (carrier oil, known for promoting hair growth)
- 2 tablespoons of jojoba oil (carrier oil, mimics the natural oils of the scalp)
- 10 drops of rosemary essential oil
- 10 drops of peppermint essential oil
- A small dropper bottle or glass container with a lid

Instructions:

1. **Prepare Your Workspace**:
   - Ensure that your dropper bottle or glass container and any mixing tools are clean and dry. Sterilizing the bottle by rinsing it with boiling water and letting it air dry can help prevent contamination.

2. **Measure and Combine Carrier Oils**:
   - o In a small bowl or directly in the dropper bottle, combine 2 tablespoons of castor oil and 2 tablespoons of jojoba oil. These carrier oils are chosen for their ability to nourish the scalp and promote hair growth.
3. **Add Essential Oils**:
   - o Add 10 drops of rosemary essential oil to the carrier oils. Rosemary oil is known for its ability to stimulate hair follicles, improve circulation, and promote hair growth.
   - o Add 10 drops of peppermint essential oil. Peppermint oil increases blood circulation to the scalp, providing a cooling sensation and promoting healthier hair follicles.
4. **Mix and Transfer**:
   - o Mix the oils thoroughly to ensure that the essential oils are evenly distributed throughout the carrier oils.
   - o Carefully transfer the mixture into your dropper bottle or glass container using a small funnel if necessary.
5. **Label and Store**:
   - o Label the dropper bottle or container with the contents and date. Store the serum in a cool, dark place to preserve the integrity of the oils. The serum should be used within six months for the best results.

Application:

- Apply a few drops of the serum to your scalp and massage gently using your fingertips. Focus on areas where you want to promote hair growth.
- Leave the serum on for at least 30 minutes before washing it out. For best results, leave it on overnight and wash your hair in the morning.
- Use the serum 2-3 times per week for optimal results.

Tips:

- For an added boost, you can warm the serum slightly before applying it to your scalp. This can help the oils penetrate more deeply.
- Perform a patch test before using the serum to ensure you don't have any allergic reactions to the essential oils.

- Consistency is key; regular use of the serum will yield the best results over time.

This Rosemary & Peppermint Hair Growth Serum harnesses the power of natural ingredients to support healthy hair growth and improve scalp health. Enjoy the invigorating sensation and the benefits of thicker, healthier hair.

17. Rosemary & Lavender Scalp Treatment

This Rosemary & Lavender Scalp Treatment is designed to nourish your scalp, promote hair growth, and soothe any irritation. Rosemary essential oil stimulates hair follicles and improves circulation, while lavender essential oil helps to calm and balance the scalp. Combined with nourishing carrier oils, this treatment will leave your scalp feeling revitalized and your hair looking healthy.

Ingredients:

- 2 tablespoons of coconut oil (moisturizing and antibacterial)
- 2 tablespoons of jojoba oil (balances sebum production and is easily absorbed)
- 10 drops of rosemary essential oil (stimulates hair follicles and improves circulation)
- 10 drops of lavender essential oil (soothes and balances the scalp)
- 1 teaspoon of vitamin E oil (optional, for added scalp benefits)
- A small glass bottle with a dropper

Instructions:

1. **Prepare Your Workspace:**
   - Ensure that your glass bottle and any mixing tools are clean and dry. Sterilizing the bottle by rinsing it with boiling water and letting it air dry can help prevent contamination.
2. **Combine Carrier Oils:**
   - In a small bowl or directly in the glass bottle, combine 2 tablespoons of coconut oil and 2 tablespoons of jojoba oil. Stir or shake well to mix.
3. **Add Essential Oils:**

    o   Add 10 drops of rosemary essential oil and 10 drops of lavender essential oil to the mixture. Essential oils should be added carefully to ensure the correct dilution and effectiveness.

4. **Add Vitamin E Oil (Optional)**:
   - If using, add 1 teaspoon of vitamin E oil to the mixture. Stir or shake well to ensure all oils are evenly distributed.

5. **Mix Thoroughly**:
   - If mixing in a bowl, stir the mixture thoroughly to ensure the essential oils are evenly distributed. If mixing directly in the glass bottle, cap the bottle and shake well to combine all ingredients.

6. **Transfer (if necessary) and Store**:
   - If you mixed the ingredients in a bowl, use a small funnel to transfer the mixture into your glass bottle. Cap the bottle tightly.

7. **Label and Store**:
   - Label the glass bottle with the contents and date. Store the scalp treatment in a cool, dark place to preserve the integrity of the oils. The treatment should be used within six months for the best results.

Application:

- Apply a few drops of the scalp treatment to your fingertips.
- Massage the treatment into your scalp using gentle, circular motions, focusing on areas that need extra care.
- Leave the treatment on for at least 30 minutes, or overnight for a more intensive treatment.
- Wash your hair with a gentle shampoo to remove the treatment.
- Use the scalp treatment once or twice a week for best results.

Tips:

- Perform a patch test before using the scalp treatment to ensure you don't have any allergic reactions to the essential oils.
- For an added cooling effect, store the scalp treatment in the refrigerator.
- Customize the scent by adjusting the essential oils to your preference, keeping the total number of drops the same.

- If you prefer a lighter treatment, reduce the amount of coconut oil and increase the amount of jojoba oil.

This Rosemary & Lavender Scalp Treatment is a luxurious enhancement to your hair care routine, offering your scalp the nourishing and stimulating benefits of premium essential oils and natural ingredients. Experience the revitalized, healthy feeling

18. Tea Tree & Rosemary Anti Dandruff Shampoo

This Tea Tree & Rosemary Anti Dandruff Shampoo is designed to help combat dandruff while soothing and nourishing the scalp. Tea tree essential oil has powerful antifungal and antibacterial properties that can help address dandruff, while rosemary essential oil stimulates hair growth and improves scalp health. Combined with a gentle, natural shampoo base, this recipe provides a refreshing and effective solution for dandruff.

Ingredients:

- 1 cup of liquid castile soap (gentle, natural shampoo base)
- 1/4 cup of distilled water (dilutes the shampoo base)
- 1 tablespoon of jojoba oil (moisturizing and nourishing for the scalp)
- 10 drops of tea tree essential oil (antifungal and antibacterial)
- 10 drops of rosemary essential oil (stimulates hair growth and improves scalp health)
- A clean shampoo bottle or squeeze bottle
- A small funnel (optional, for easier pouring)

Instructions:

1. **Prepare Your Workspace:**
   - Ensure that your shampoo bottle and any mixing tools are clean and dry. Sterilizing the bottle by rinsing it with boiling water and letting it air dry can help prevent contamination.
2. **Combine Liquid Ingredients:**
   - In a small bowl or directly in the shampoo bottle, combine 1 cup of liquid castile soap and 1/4 cup of distilled water. Stir or shake well to mix.
3. **Add Jojoba Oil:**

- o Add 1 tablespoon of jojoba oil to the liquid mixture. Jojoba oil is known for its moisturizing and nourishing properties, which can help soothe the scalp.

4. **Add Essential Oils**:
   - o Add 10 drops of tea tree essential oil and 10 drops of rosemary essential oil to the mixture. Essential oils should be added carefully to ensure the correct dilution and effectiveness.

5. **Mix Thoroughly**:
   - o If mixing in a bowl, stir the mixture thoroughly to ensure the essential oils and jojoba oil are evenly distributed. If mixing directly in the shampoo bottle, cap the bottle and shake well to combine all ingredients.

6. **Transfer (if necessary) and Store**:
   - o If you mixed the ingredients in a bowl, use a small funnel to transfer the mixture into your shampoo bottle. Cap the bottle tightly.

7. **Label and Store**:
   - o Label the bottle with the contents and date. Store the shampoo in a cool, dark place to preserve the integrity of the ingredients. The shampoo should be used within six months for the best results.

Application:

- Wet your hair thoroughly with warm water.
- Apply a small amount of the Tea Tree & Rosemary Anti Dandruff Shampoo to your scalp and hair.
- Gently massage the shampoo into your scalp using your fingertips, focusing on areas with dandruff.
- Rinse thoroughly with warm water and follow with your regular conditioner if desired.
- Use the shampoo 2-3 times a week for best results.

Tips:

- Perform a patch test before using the shampoo to ensure you don't have any allergic reactions to the essential oils.

- Shake the bottle well before each use to ensure the essential oils are evenly distributed.
- Customize the scent by adjusting the essential oils to your preference, keeping the total number of drops the same.
- For an added cooling effect, store the shampoo in the refrigerator.

This Tea Tree & Rosemary Anti Dandruff Shampoo is wonderful at providing your scalp with the antifungal and antibacterial benefits of tea tree oil and the stimulating properties of rosemary oil. Enjoy the refreshing, soothing experience and a healthy, dandruff-free scalp.

19. Jasmine & Sandalwood Hair Perfume

This Jasmine & Sandalwood Hair Perfume is designed to add a luxurious fragrance to your hair while providing some conditioning benefits. Jasmine essential oil offers a sweet, floral scent and promotes hair softness, while sandalwood essential oil has a warm, woody aroma and helps to condition the scalp. Combined with a lightweight carrier oil and water, this hair perfume will leave your hair smelling divine and feeling smooth.

Ingredients:

- 1/4 cup of distilled water (base for the perfume)
- 2 tablespoons of rose water (adds a subtle floral scent and benefits the scalp)
- 1 teaspoon of jojoba oil (lightweight and moisturizing)
- 10 drops of jasmine essential oil (sweet, floral scent and promotes hair softness)
- 5 drops of sandalwood essential oil (warm, woody aroma and conditions the scalp)
- A small spray bottle (preferably glass)
- A small funnel (optional, for easier pouring)

Instructions:

1. **Prepare Your Workspace:**
   - Ensure that your spray bottle and any mixing tools are clean and dry. Sterilizing the bottle by rinsing it with boiling water and letting it air dry can help prevent contamination.
2. **Combine Liquid Ingredients:**
   - In a small bowl or directly in the spray bottle, combine 1/4 cup of distilled water and 2 tablespoons of rose water. Stir or shake well to mix.
3. **Add Jojoba Oil:**

o   Add 1 teaspoon of jojoba oil to the liquid mixture. Jojoba oil is lightweight and provides moisturizing benefits without weighing down your hair.

4. **Add Essential Oils**:
   o   Add 10 drops of jasmine essential oil and 5 drops of sandalwood essential oil to the mixture. Essential oils should be added carefully to ensure the correct dilution and effectiveness.

5. **Mix Thoroughly**:
   o   If mixing in a bowl, stir the mixture thoroughly to ensure the essential oils and jojoba oil are evenly distributed. If mixing directly in the spray bottle, cap the bottle and shake well to combine all ingredients.

6. **Transfer (if necessary) and Store**:
   o   If you mixed the ingredients in a bowl, use a small funnel to transfer the mixture into your spray bottle. Cap the bottle tightly.

7. **Label and Store**:
   o   Label the spray bottle with the contents and date. Store the hair perfume in a cool, dark place to preserve the integrity of the ingredients. The hair perfume should be used within six months for the best results.

Application:

- Hold the spray bottle about 6-8 inches away from your hair.
- Lightly mist the hair perfume over your hair, focusing on the mid-lengths to ends.
- Avoid spraying directly on the scalp to prevent oil buildup.
- Use the hair perfume as needed to refresh the scent of your hair throughout the day.

Tips:

- Perform a patch test before using the hair perfume to ensure you don't have any allergic reactions to the essential oils.
- Shake the bottle well before each use to ensure the essential oils are evenly distributed.

- Customize the scent by adjusting the essential oils to your preference, keeping the total number of drops the same.
- For a stronger scent, increase the number of drops of essential oils, maintaining the same ratio. 53

This Jasmine & Sandalwood Hair Perfume is a luxurious addition to your hair care routine, providing your hair with a beautiful fragrance and some conditioning benefits. Enjoy the sweet, floral, and woody scent that follows you throughout the day.

5. ESSENTIAL OIL RECIPES FOR THE BODY

20. Orange & Vanilla Body Scrub

This Orange & Vanilla Body Scrub is a delightful and luxurious addition to your skincare routine. The zesty orange essential oil invigorates the senses and promotes a radiant complexion, while vanilla essential oil provides a warm, comforting aroma and helps soothe the skin. Combined with exfoliating sugar and moisturizing oils, this body scrub will leave your skin feeling soft, smooth, and refreshed.

Ingredients:

- 1 cup of granulated sugar (exfoliates and removes dead skin cells)
- 1/2 cup of coconut oil (moisturizes and nourishes the skin)
- 1 teaspoon of vanilla extract (soothes and provides a comforting aroma)
- 10 drops of orange essential oil (invigorates and brightens the skin)
- 1 tablespoon of sweet almond oil (optional, for added hydration)
- A small mixing bowl
- A spoon or spatula for mixing
- A clean glass jar or container with a lid

Instructions:

1. **Prepare Your Workspace**:
   - o Ensure that your glass jar or container and any mixing tools are clean and dry. Sterilizing the jar by rinsing it with boiling water and letting it air dry can help prevent contamination.
2. **Combine Sugar and Oils**:
   - o In a small mixing bowl, combine 1 cup of granulated sugar with 1/2 cup of coconut oil. If using, add 1 tablespoon of sweet almond oil. Mix well until the sugar is evenly coated with the oils.
3. **Add Vanilla Extract and Essential Oil**:
   - o Add 1 teaspoon of vanilla extract and 10 drops of orange essential oil to the mixture. Stir thoroughly to ensure the extract and essential oil are evenly distributed.
4. **Mix Thoroughly**:
   - o Using a spoon or spatula, continue to mix the scrub until all ingredients are well combined and the texture is consistent.
5. **Transfer and Store**:
   - o Carefully transfer the body scrub into your clean glass jar or container using a spoon or spatula. Ensure the jar is filled and sealed tightly with a lid.
6. **Label and Store**:
   - o Label the jar with the contents and date. Store the body scrub in a cool, dark place to preserve the integrity of the oils and sugars. The body scrub should be used within three months for the best results.

Application:

- In the shower or bath, apply a small amount of the body scrub to damp skin.
- Gently massage the scrub in circular motions, focusing on areas that need extra exfoliation, such as elbows, knees, and feet.
- Rinse thoroughly with warm water and pat your skin dry.
- Use the body scrub 1-2 times a week for best results.

Tips:

- Perform a patch test before using the body scrub to ensure you don't have any allergic reactions to the essential oils.

- Customize the scent by adjusting the essential oils to your preference, keeping the total number of drops the same.
- For a coarser scrub, increase the amount of sugar; for a gentler scrub, reduce the amount of sugar and add more oil.
- If the scrub hardens, place the jar in warm water to soften the coconut oil before use.

This Orange & Vanilla Body Scrub is a delightful way to pamper your skin, providing exfoliation and moisture with the invigorating scent of orange and the comforting aroma of vanilla. Enjoy soft, smooth, and refreshed skin.

21. Orange & Cinnamon Energizing Body Wash

This Orange & Cinnamon Energizing Body Wash is designed to invigorate your senses and refresh your skin. Orange essential oil revitalizes and brightens the skin, while cinnamon essential oil provides a warm, stimulating effect. Combined with a gentle cleansing base, this body wash will leave your skin feeling clean, soft, and energized.

Ingredients:

- 1/2 cup of liquid castile soap (gentle and natural cleanser)
- 1/4 cup of distilled water
- 1 tablespoon of sweet almond oil (moisturizing and nourishing)
- 1 teaspoon of vegetable glycerin (optional, for added moisture)
- 15 drops of orange essential oil (revitalizes and brightens the skin)
- 5 drops of cinnamon essential oil (stimulating and warming)
- A small mixing bowl
- A clean pump bottle or squeeze bottle

Instructions:

1. **Prepare Your Workspace:**
   - Ensure that your pump bottle or squeeze bottle and any mixing tools are clean and dry. Sterilizing the bottle by rinsing it with boiling water and letting it air dry can help prevent contamination.
2. **Combine Liquid Ingredients:**
   - In a small mixing bowl, combine 1/2 cup of liquid castile soap, 1/4 cup of distilled water, 1 tablespoon of sweet almond oil, and 1 teaspoon of vegetable glycerin (if using). Stir well to mix.
3. **Add Essential Oils:**

    o   Add 15 drops of orange essential oil and 5 drops of cinnamon essential oil to the mixture. Stir thoroughly to ensure the essential oils are evenly distributed.

4. **Mix Thoroughly**:
   - Continue to stir the mixture until all ingredients are well combined and the texture is consistent.

5. **Transfer and Store**:
   - Carefully transfer the body wash into your clean pump bottle or squeeze bottle using a funnel if needed. Ensure the bottle is filled and sealed tightly with a lid.

6. **Label and Store**:
   - Label the bottle with the contents and date. Store the body wash in a cool, dark place to preserve the integrity of the ingredients. The body wash should be used within three months for the best results.

Application:

- In the shower or bath, apply a small amount of the body wash to a washcloth, loofah, or your hands.
- Gently lather the body wash onto your skin, using circular motions to cleanse and invigorate.
- Rinse thoroughly with warm water and pat your skin dry.
- Use the body wash daily for an energizing and refreshing start to your day.

Tips:

- Perform a patch test before using the body wash to ensure you don't have any allergic reactions to the essential oils.
- Customize the scent by adjusting the essential oils to your preference, keeping the total number of drops the same.
- For a thicker consistency, add a small amount of xanthan gum and mix well.
- If you prefer a more moisturizing body wash, increase the amount of sweet almond oil slightly.

This Orange & Cinnamon Energizing Body Wash is a delightful way to start your day, providing your skin with a refreshing cleanse and an invigorating feel.

22. Ylang Ylang & Geranium Moisturizing Lotion

This Ylang Ylang & Geranium Moisturizing Lotion is designed to hydrate and nourish your skin while leaving a delicate, floral scent. Ylang ylang essential oil helps balance skin oil production, while geranium essential oil provides anti-inflammatory and antiseptic benefits. Combined with rich carrier oils and butters, this lotion will keep your skin soft and smooth.

Ingredients:

- 1/4 cup of shea butter (deeply moisturizing and rich in vitamins A and E)
- 1/4 cup of coconut oil (hydrates and protects the skin)
- 1/4 cup of sweet almond oil (lightweight and easily absorbed)
- 1/4 cup of aloe vera gel (soothing and hydrating)
- 10 drops of ylang ylang essential oil (balancing and soothing)
- 10 drops of geranium essential oil (anti-inflammatory and antiseptic)
- 1 teaspoon of vitamin E oil (optional, for added antioxidant benefits)
- A double boiler or heat-safe bowl and saucepan
- A hand mixer or whisk
- A clean glass jar or container with a lid

Instructions:

1. **Prepare Your Workspace:**
    - Ensure that your glass jar or container and any mixing tools are clean and dry. Sterilizing the jar by rinsing it with boiling water and letting it air dry can help prevent contamination.
2. **Melt the Shea Butter and Coconut Oil:**
    - In a double boiler or a heat-safe bowl set over a saucepan of simmering water, melt 1/4 cup of shea butter and 1/4 cup of coconut oil. Stir occasionally until fully melted and combined.

3. **Add Sweet Almond Oil and Aloe Vera Gel**:
   - o Remove the melted shea butter and coconut oil from heat. Add 1/4 cup of sweet almond oil and 1/4 cup of aloe vera gel to the mixture. Stir well to combine.

4. **Incorporate Essential Oils**:
   - o Allow the mixture to cool slightly but not solidify. Add 10 drops of ylang ylang essential oil and 10 drops of geranium essential oil to the mixture. If using, add 1 teaspoon of vitamin E oil for its additional antioxidant benefits.

5. **Mix and Whip**:
   - o Using a hand mixer or whisk, blend the mixture until it becomes creamy and smooth. This may take a few minutes and will help to create a light, whipped texture for the lotion.

6. **Transfer and Store**:
   - o Carefully transfer the whipped lotion into your glass jar or container using a spatula. Ensure the jar is filled and sealed tightly with a lid.

7. **Label and Store**:
   - o Label the jar with the contents and date. Store the lotion in a cool, dark place to preserve the integrity of the oils and butters. The lotion should be used within six months for the best results.

Application:

- Apply a small amount of the lotion to clean, dry skin. Focus on areas that need extra hydration, such as hands, elbows, and knees.
- Gently massage the lotion into your skin using upward, circular motions until fully absorbed.
- Use the lotion daily for soft, smooth, and hydrated skin.

Tips:

- For an added cooling effect, store the lotion in the refrigerator.
- Perform a patch test before using the lotion to ensure you don't have any allergic reactions to the essential oils.
- Customize the scent by adjusting the essential oils to your preference, keeping the total number of drops the same.

This Ylang Ylang & Geranium Moisturizing Lotion, provides your skin with the hydrating and balancing benefits of high-quality essential oils and nourishing butters. Enjoy the floral aroma and the silky, smooth skin.

61

23. Jasmine & Vanilla Body Butter

This Jasmine & Vanilla Body Butter is a rich and luxurious moisturizer that deeply nourishes the skin. Jasmine essential oil provides a delightful floral scent and promotes relaxation, while vanilla extract adds a warm, comforting aroma. The combination of shea butter, coconut oil, and sweet almond oil ensures that your skin stays soft and hydrated.

Ingredients:

- 1/2 cup of shea butter (deeply moisturizing and rich in vitamins A and E)
- 1/4 cup of coconut oil (hydrates and protects the skin)
- 1/4 cup of sweet almond oil (lightweight and easily absorbed)
- 10 drops of jasmine essential oil (relaxing and fragrant)
- 1 teaspoon of vanilla extract (warm and comforting aroma)
- A double boiler or heat-safe bowl and saucepan
- A hand mixer or whisk
- A clean glass jar or container with a lid

Instructions:

1. **Prepare Your Workspace:**
   - Ensure that your glass jar or container and any mixing tools are clean and dry. Sterilizing the jar by rinsing it with boiling water and letting it air dry can help prevent contamination.
2. **Melt the Shea Butter and Coconut Oil:**
   - In a double boiler or a heat-safe bowl set over a saucepan of simmering water, melt 1/2 cup of shea butter and 1/4 cup of coconut oil. Stir occasionally until fully melted and combined.
3. **Add Sweet Almond Oil:**
   - Remove the melted shea butter and coconut oil from heat. Add 1/4 cup of sweet almond oil to the mixture and stir well to combine.

4. **Cool Slightly and Add Essential Oils**:
   - o Allow the mixture to cool slightly but not solidify. Add 10 drops of jasmine essential oil and 1 teaspoon of vanilla extract. Stir well to ensure the essential oils and extract are evenly distributed.
5. **Mix and Whip**:
   - o Using a hand mixer or whisk, blend the mixture until it becomes creamy and smooth. This may take a few minutes and will help to create a light, whipped texture for the body butter.
6. **Transfer and Store**:
   - o Carefully transfer the whipped body butter into your glass jar or container using a spatula. Ensure the jar is filled and sealed tightly with a lid.
7. **Label and Store**:
   - o Label the jar with the contents and date. Store the body butter in a cool, dark place to preserve the integrity of the oils and butters. The body butter should be used within six months for the best results.

Application:

- Apply a small amount of the body butter to clean, dry skin. Focus on areas that need extra hydration, such as hands, elbows, and knees.
- Gently massage the body butter into your skin using upward, circular motions until fully absorbed.
- Use the body butter daily for soft, smooth, and hydrated skin.

Tips:

- Perform a patch test before using the body butter to ensure you don't have any allergic reactions to the essential oils.
- For an added cooling effect, store the body butter in the refrigerator.
- Customize the scent by adjusting the essential oils to your preference, keeping the total number of drops the same.
- If you prefer a firmer body butter, increase the amount of shea butter slightly.

This Jasmine & Vanilla Body Butter gives your skin nourishment and hydration. Enjoy the rich, comforting aroma and the soft, smooth skin that follows.

24. Bergamot & Lavender After Shaving Balm

This Bergamot & Lavender After Shaving Balm is designed to soothe and moisturize your skin after shaving. Bergamot essential oil has antiseptic and calming properties, while lavender essential oil helps to soothe irritation and reduce redness. Combined with nourishing carrier oils and butters, this aftershave balm will leave your skin feeling soft, smooth, and refreshed.

Ingredients:

- 1/4 cup of shea butter (deeply moisturizing and rich in vitamins A and E)
- 2 tablespoons of coconut oil (hydrates and protects the skin)
- 2 tablespoons of sweet almond oil (lightweight and easily absorbed)
- 10 drops of bergamot essential oil (antiseptic and calming)
- 10 drops of lavender essential oil (soothing and anti-inflammatory)
- 1 teaspoon of vitamin E oil (optional, for added skin benefits)
- A double boiler or heat-safe bowl and saucepan
- A hand mixer or whisk
- A clean glass jar or container with a lid

Instructions:

1. **Prepare Your Workspace**:
    - Ensure that your glass jar or container and any mixing tools are clean and dry. Sterilizing the jar by rinsing it with boiling water and letting it air dry can help prevent contamination.
2. **Melt the Shea Butter and Coconut Oil**:

- o In a double boiler or a heat-safe bowl set over a saucepan of simmering water, melt 1/4 cup of shea butter and 2 tablespoons of coconut oil. Stir occasionally until fully melted and combined.
3. **Add Sweet Almond Oil**:
    - o Remove the melted shea butter and coconut oil from heat. Add 2 tablespoons of sweet almond oil to the mixture and stir well to combine.
4. **Cool Slightly and Add Essential Oils**:
    - o Allow the mixture to cool slightly but not solidify. Add 10 drops of bergamot essential oil and 10 drops of lavender essential oil. If using, add 1 teaspoon of vitamin E oil. Stir well to ensure the essential oils and vitamin E oil are evenly distributed.
5. **Mix and Whip**:
    - o Using a hand mixer or whisk, blend the mixture until it becomes creamy and smooth. This may take a few minutes and will help to create a light, whipped texture for the aftershave balm.
6. **Transfer and Store**:
    - o Carefully transfer the whipped aftershave balm into your glass jar or container using a spatula. Ensure the jar is filled and sealed tightly with a lid.
7. **Label and Store**:
    - o Label the jar with the contents and date. Store the aftershave balm in a cool, dark place to preserve the integrity of the oils and butters. The aftershave balm should be used within six months for the best results.

Application:

- After shaving, apply a small amount of the balm to your legs and other areas
- Gently massage the balm into your skin until fully absorbed.
- Use the after shaving balm as needed to soothe and moisturize your skin.

Tips:

- Perform a patch test before using the after shaving balm to ensure you don't have any allergic reactions to the essential oils.
- For an added cooling effect, store the after shaving balm in the refrigerator.

- Customize the scent by adjusting the essential oils to your preference, keeping the total number of drops the same.
- If you prefer a firmer balm, increase the amount of shea butter slightly.

This Bergamot & Lavender After Shaving Balm is a luxurious addition to your post-shave routine, offering your skin the soothing and moisturizing benefits of premium essential oils and natural ingredients. Indulge in the smooth, refreshed sensation.

25. Grapefruit & Cypress Cellulite Cream

This Grapefruit & Cypress Cellulite Cream is designed to help reduce the appearance of cellulite by improving circulation and tightening the skin. Grapefruit essential oil has detoxifying properties that can help break down fat cells, while cypress essential oil improves circulation and has a toning effect. Combined with moisturizing shea butter and coconut oil, this cream will leave your skin feeling smooth and firm.

Ingredients:

- 1/4 cup of shea butter (deeply moisturizing and rich in vitamins A and E)
- 2 tablespoons of coconut oil (hydrates and protects the skin)
- 2 tablespoons of jojoba oil (lightweight and easily absorbed)
- 10 drops of grapefruit essential oil (detoxifying and fat cell breakdown)
- 10 drops of cypress essential oil (improves circulation and tones skin)
- 1 teaspoon of vitamin E oil (optional, for added skin benefits)
- A double boiler or heat-safe bowl and saucepan
- A hand mixer or whisk
- A clean glass jar or container with a lid

Instructions:

1. **Prepare Your Workspace**:
   - Ensure that your glass jar or container and any mixing tools are clean and dry. Sterilizing the jar by rinsing it with boiling water and letting it air dry can help prevent contamination.
2. **Melt the Shea Butter and Coconut Oil**:
   - In a double boiler or a heat-safe bowl set over a saucepan of simmering water, melt 1/4 cup of shea butter and 2 tablespoons of coconut oil. Stir occasionally until fully melted and combined.
3. **Add Jojoba Oil**:

- o   Remove the melted shea butter and coconut oil from heat. Add 2 tablespoons of jojoba oil to the mixture and stir well to combine.

4.   **Cool Slightly and Add Essential Oils**:
   - o   Allow the mixture to cool slightly but not solidify. Add 10 drops of grapefruit essential oil and 10 drops of cypress essential oil. If using, add 1 teaspoon of vitamin E oil. Stir well to ensure the essential oils and vitamin E oil are evenly distributed.

5.   **Mix and Whip**:
   - o   Using a hand mixer or whisk, blend the mixture until it becomes creamy and smooth. This may take a few minutes and will help to create a light, whipped texture for the cellulite cream.

6.   **Transfer and Store**:
   - o   Carefully transfer the whipped cellulite cream into your glass jar or container using a spatula. Ensure the jar is filled and sealed tightly with a lid.

7.   **Label and Store**:
   - o   Label the jar with the contents and date. Store the cellulite cream in a cool, dark place to preserve the integrity of the oils and butters. The cream should be used within six months for the best results.

Application:

- Apply a small amount of the cellulite cream to clean, dry skin, focusing on areas with cellulite.
- Gently massage the cream into your skin using firm, circular motions to help improve circulation and absorption.
- Use the cellulite cream daily, preferably after a shower or bath, for best results.

Tips:

- Perform a patch test before using the cellulite cream to ensure you don't have any allergic reactions to the essential oils.
- For an added cooling effect, store the cellulite cream in the refrigerator.
- Customize the scent by adjusting the essential oils to your preference, keeping the total number of drops the same.

- If you prefer a firmer cellulite cream, increase the amount of shea butter slightly.

This Grapefruit & Cypress Cellulite Cream, provides your skin with detoxifying and toning benefits to give smooth and firm skin.

6. ESSENTIAL OIL RECIPES FOR PAMPER TIME

26. Eucalyptus & Lemon Foot Scrub

This invigorating Eucalyptus & Lemon Foot Scrub is perfect for exfoliating and refreshing tired feet. Eucalyptus essential oil has cooling and antiseptic properties, while lemon essential oil brightens and revitalizes the skin. Combined with exfoliating sugar and moisturizing coconut oil, this foot scrub will leave your feet feeling soft and rejuvenated.

Ingredients:

- 1 cup of granulated sugar (exfoliating agent)
- 1/2 cup of coconut oil (moisturizing and nourishing)
- 10 drops of eucalyptus essential oil (cooling and antiseptic)
- 10 drops of lemon essential oil (brightening and revitalizing)
- 1 tablespoon of lemon zest (optional, for added fragrance and exfoliation)
- A small mixing bowl
- A clean glass jar or container with a lid

Instructions:

1. **Prepare Your Workspace**:
   - o Ensure that your glass jar or container and any mixing tools are clean and dry. Sterilizing the jar by rinsing it with boiling water and letting it air dry can help prevent contamination.
2. **Combine Sugar and Coconut Oil**:
   - o In a small mixing bowl, combine 1 cup of granulated sugar and 1/2 cup of coconut oil. Mix thoroughly until the sugar is evenly coated with the oil. The coconut oil should be in a semi-solid state; if it's too solid, you can soften it slightly by warming it in a microwave or over a double boiler.
3. **Add Essential Oils**:
   - o Add 10 drops of eucalyptus essential oil to the sugar and coconut oil mixture. Eucalyptus oil provides a refreshing, cooling sensation and has antiseptic properties that help keep your feet clean.
   - o Add 10 drops of lemon essential oil. Lemon oil brightens and revitalizes the skin, giving the scrub a refreshing citrus scent.
4. **Optional: Add Lemon Zest**:
   - o For added fragrance and exfoliation, mix in 1 tablespoon of lemon zest. The zest adds a natural, fresh lemon scent and provides additional texture for exfoliation.
5. **Mix Thoroughly**:
   - o Stir the mixture until all the ingredients are well combined and the essential oils are evenly distributed throughout the sugar and coconut oil.
6. **Transfer and Store**:
   - o Carefully transfer the foot scrub into your glass jar or container using a spatula. Ensure the jar is filled and sealed tightly with a lid.
7. **Label and Store**:
   - o Label the jar with the contents and date. Store the scrub in a cool, dark place to preserve the integrity of the oils. The scrub should be used within six months for the best results.

Application:

- Apply a small amount of the foot scrub to damp feet, focusing on rough or calloused areas.

- Gently massage the scrub into your skin using circular motions to exfoliate and refresh your feet.
- Rinse thoroughly with warm water and pat dry.
- Use the foot scrub 1-2 times a week for soft, smooth, and revitalized feet.

Tips:

- Perform a patch test before using the scrub to ensure you don't have any allergic reactions to the essential oils.
- For an added cooling effect, store the scrub in the refrigerator.
- Be cautious when using the scrub in the shower or bathtub, as the coconut oil can make surfaces slippery.

This Eucalyptus & Lemon Foot Scrub is a delightful addition to your foot care routine, providing your feet with the exfoliating and refreshing benefits of high-quality essential oils and natural ingredients. Enjoy the invigorating sensation and the smooth, revitalized feet that follow.

27. Geranium & Lemon Cuticle Oil

This Geranium & Lemon Cuticle Oil is designed to nourish and strengthen your cuticles and nails. Geranium essential oil promotes healthy skin and nail growth, while lemon essential oil helps brighten and strengthen nails. Combined with nourishing carrier oils, this cuticle oil will keep your nails looking healthy and beautiful.

Ingredients:

- 2 tablespoons of jojoba oil (moisturizing and easily absorbed)
- 1 tablespoon of sweet almond oil (nourishing and hydrating)
- 1 tablespoon of vitamin E oil (strengthens nails and promotes healthy cuticles)
- 10 drops of geranium essential oil (promotes healthy skin and nail growth)
- 10 drops of lemon essential oil (brightens and strengthens nails)
- A small glass dropper bottle
- A small funnel (optional, for easier pouring)

Instructions:

1. **Prepare Your Workspace:**
   - Ensure that your dropper bottle and any mixing tools are clean and dry. Sterilizing the bottle by rinsing it with boiling water and letting it air dry can help prevent contamination.
2. **Combine Carrier Oils:**
   - In a small bowl or directly in the dropper bottle, combine 2 tablespoons of jojoba oil, 1 tablespoon of sweet almond oil, and 1 tablespoon of vitamin E oil. Stir or shake well to mix.
3. **Add Essential Oils:**

o   Add 10 drops of geranium essential oil and 10 drops of lemon essential oil to the mixture. Essential oils should be added carefully to ensure the correct dilution and effectiveness.

4. **Mix Thoroughly**:
    o   If mixing in a bowl, stir the mixture thoroughly to ensure the essential oils are evenly distributed. If mixing directly in the dropper bottle, cap the bottle and shake well to combine all ingredients.

5. **Transfer (if necessary) and Store**:
    o   If you mixed the ingredients in a bowl, use a small funnel to transfer the mixture into your dropper bottle. Cap the bottle tightly.

6. **Label and Store**:
    o   Label the dropper bottle with the contents and date. Store the cuticle oil in a cool, dark place to preserve the integrity of the oils. The cuticle oil should be used within six months for the best results.

Application:

- Apply a small drop of the cuticle oil to each nail.
- Gently massage the oil into your cuticles and nails using your fingertips.
- Use the cuticle oil daily or as needed to keep your cuticles and nails healthy and hydrated.

Tips:

- Perform a patch test before using the cuticle oil to ensure you don't have any allergic reactions to the essential oils.
- For an added cooling effect, store the cuticle oil in the refrigerator.
- Customize the scent by adjusting the essential oils to your preference, keeping the total number of drops the same.
- If you prefer a lighter oil, reduce the amount of vitamin E oil slightly and increase the amount of jojoba or sweet almond oil.

This Geranium & Lemon Cuticle Oil, gives your cuticles and nails nourishment and strength. Enjoy the healthy and beautiful nails

28. Lemon & Basil Hand Cream

This Lemon & Basil Hand Cream is designed to nourish and hydrate your hands while providing a refreshing and uplifting scent. Lemon essential oil offers brightening and antiseptic properties, while basil essential oil provides a soothing and calming effect. Combined with rich shea butter and moisturizing oils, this hand cream will leave your hands feeling soft and rejuvenated.

Ingredients:

- 1/4 cup of shea butter (deeply moisturizing and rich in vitamins A and E)
- 2 tablespoons of coconut oil (hydrates and protects the skin)
- 2 tablespoons of sweet almond oil (lightweight and easily absorbed)
- 10 drops of lemon essential oil (brightening and antiseptic)
- 5 drops of basil essential oil (soothing and calming)
- 1 teaspoon of vitamin E oil (optional, for added skin benefits)
- A double boiler or heat-safe bowl and saucepan
- A hand mixer or whisk
- A clean glass jar or container with a lid

Instructions:

1. **Prepare Your Workspace**:
   - Ensure that your glass jar or container and any mixing tools are clean and dry. Sterilizing the jar by rinsing it with boiling water and letting it air dry can help prevent contamination.
2. **Melt the Shea Butter and Coconut Oil**:
   - In a double boiler or a heat-safe bowl set over a saucepan of simmering water, melt 1/4 cup of shea butter and 2 tablespoons of coconut oil. Stir occasionally until fully melted and combined.
3. **Add Sweet Almond Oil**:

- o Remove the melted shea butter and coconut oil from heat. Add 2 tablespoons of sweet almond oil to the mixture and stir well to combine.

4. **Cool Slightly and Add Essential Oils**:
   - o Allow the mixture to cool slightly but not solidify. Add 10 drops of lemon essential oil and 5 drops of basil essential oil. If using, add 1 teaspoon of vitamin E oil. Stir well to ensure the essential oils and vitamin E oil are evenly distributed.

5. **Mix and Whip**:
   - o Using a hand mixer or whisk, blend the mixture until it becomes creamy and smooth. This may take a few minutes and will help to create a light, whipped texture for the hand cream.

6. **Transfer and Store**:
   - o Carefully transfer the whipped hand cream into your glass jar or container using a spatula. Ensure the jar is filled and sealed tightly with a lid.

7. **Label and Store**:
   - o Label the jar with the contents and date. Store the hand cream in a cool, dark place to preserve the integrity of the oils and butters. The hand cream should be used within six months for the best results.

Application:

- Apply a small amount of the hand cream to clean, dry hands.
- Gently massage the cream into your hands, focusing on areas that need extra hydration, such as knuckles and cuticles.
- Use the hand cream as needed throughout the day for soft, smooth hands.

Tips:

- Perform a patch test before using the hand cream to ensure you don't have any allergic reactions to the essential oils.
- For an added cooling effect, store the hand cream in the refrigerator.
- Customize the scent by adjusting the essential oils to your preference, keeping the total number of drops the same.
- If you prefer a firmer hand cream, increase the amount of shea butter slightly.

This Lemon & Basil Hand Cream is a luxurious, providing your hands with the nourishing and hydrating benefits of high-quality essential oils and butters. Enjoy the refreshing, uplifting scent and soft, rejuvenated hands.

77

29. Clary Sage & Lavender Relaxing Bath Soak

This Clary Sage & Lavender Relaxing Bath Soak is perfect for unwinding after a long day. Clary sage essential oil helps to reduce stress and promote relaxation, while lavender essential oil soothes the mind and body. Combined with Epsom salts, this bath soak will leave you feeling calm and rejuvenated.

Ingredients:

- 1 cup of Epsom salts (relieves muscle tension and detoxifies the body)
- 1/2 cup of sea salt (softens the skin and helps to cleanse)
- 1/2 cup of baking soda (soothes irritated skin and neutralizes acids)
- 10 drops of clary sage essential oil (reduces stress and promotes relaxation)
- 10 drops of lavender essential oil (soothes the mind and body)
- 1 tablespoon of dried lavender flowers (optional, for added fragrance and aesthetics)
- 1 tablespoon of dried sage leaves (optional, for added fragrance and aesthetics)
- A large mixing bowl
- An airtight container or jar

Instructions:

1. **Prepare Your Workspace**:
   - Ensure that your mixing bowl and any tools are clean and dry. Sterilizing the container by rinsing it with boiling water and letting it air dry can help prevent contamination.
2. **Combine the Dry Ingredients**:
   - In a large mixing bowl, combine 1 cup of Epsom salts, 1/2 cup of sea salt, and 1/2 cup of baking soda. Mix thoroughly until the dry ingredients are evenly distributed.

3. **Add Essential Oils**:
   - o   Add 10 drops of clary sage essential oil and 10 drops of lavender essential oil to the dry mixture. Stir well to ensure the essential oils are evenly distributed throughout the salts.
4. **Optional: Add Dried Flowers and Leaves**:
   - o   For added fragrance and aesthetics, mix in 1 tablespoon of dried lavender flowers and 1 tablespoon of dried sage leaves. These ingredients are optional but can enhance the relaxing experience.
5. **Mix Thoroughly**:
   - o   Stir the mixture until all the ingredients are well combined. Ensure that the essential oils are evenly distributed to prevent clumping.
6. **Transfer and Store**:
   - o   Carefully transfer the bath soak mixture into your airtight container or jar using a funnel if necessary. Seal the container tightly to keep the bath soak fresh.
7. **Label and Store**:
   - o   Label the container with the contents and date. Store the bath soak in a cool, dry place to preserve the integrity of the ingredients. The bath soak should be used within six months for the best results.

Application:

- Fill your bathtub with warm water.
- Add 1/2 to 1 cup of the Clary Sage & Lavender Bath Soak to the water and stir to dissolve.
- Soak in the bath for at least 20 minutes to allow the ingredients to work their magic.
- Relax and enjoy the calming, soothing effects of the bath soak.

Tips:

- Perform a patch test before using the bath soak to ensure you don't have any allergic reactions to the essential oils.
- Store the bath soak in an airtight container to keep it fresh and prevent the essential oils from evaporating.
- Customize the scent by adjusting the essential oils to your preference, keeping the total number of drops the same.

This Clary Sage & Lavender Relaxing Bath Soak, provides your body and mind with the soothing and calming benefits of high-quality essential oils and natural ingredients. Enjoy the tranquil, rejuvenating experience and the peaceful sleep that follows.

30. Lavender & Tea Tree Deodorant

This Lavender & Tea Tree Deodorant is a natural, effective solution to keep you feeling fresh and odor-free. Lavender essential oil has soothing and antibacterial properties, while tea tree essential oil provides strong antimicrobial benefits. Combined with coconut oil, shea butter, and baking soda, this deodorant is gentle on the skin and provides long-lasting protection.

Ingredients:

- 1/4 cup of coconut oil (antibacterial and moisturizing)
- 1/4 cup of shea butter (soothing and nourishing)
- 1/4 cup of arrowroot powder (absorbs moisture)
- 1/4 cup of baking soda (neutralizes odor)
- 10 drops of lavender essential oil (soothing and antibacterial)
- 10 drops of tea tree essential oil (antimicrobial and deodorizing)
- A double boiler or heat-safe bowl and saucepan
- A hand mixer or whisk
- A clean, empty deodorant container or small glass jar with a lid

Instructions:

1. **Prepare Your Workspace**:
   - Ensure that your deodorant container or jar and any mixing tools are clean and dry. Sterilizing the container by rinsing it with boiling water and letting it air dry can help prevent contamination.
2. **Melt the Coconut Oil and Shea Butter**:
   - In a double boiler or a heat-safe bowl set over a saucepan of simmering water, melt 1/4 cup of coconut oil and 1/4 cup of shea butter. Stir occasionally until fully melted and combined.
3. **Add Arrowroot Powder and Baking Soda**:

o   Remove the melted coconut oil and shea butter from heat. Add 1/4 cup of arrowroot powder and 1/4 cup of baking soda to the mixture. Stir well to combine until a smooth paste forms.

4. **Add Essential Oils**:
    o   Allow the mixture to cool slightly but not solidify. Add 10 drops of lavender essential oil and 10 drops of tea tree essential oil. Stir well to ensure the essential oils are evenly distributed.

5. **Mix Thoroughly**:
    o   Using a hand mixer or whisk, blend the mixture until it becomes creamy and smooth. This may take a few minutes and will help to create a uniform consistency for the deodorant.

6. **Transfer and Store**:
    o   Carefully transfer the deodorant mixture into your deodorant container or small glass jar using a spatula. Ensure the container is filled and sealed tightly with a lid.

7. **Label and Store**:
    o   Label the container with the contents and date. Store the deodorant in a cool, dark place to preserve the integrity of the oils and powders. The deodorant should be used within six months for the best results.

Application:

- Apply a small amount of the deodorant to clean, dry underarms.
- Gently massage the deodorant into your skin until fully absorbed.
- Use the deodorant daily or as needed to stay fresh and odor-free.

Tips:

- Perform a patch test before using the deodorant to ensure you don't have any allergic reactions to the essential oils.
- For a firmer deodorant, store the container in the refrigerator.
- Customize the scent by adjusting the essential oils to your preference, keeping the total number of drops the same.
- If you prefer a softer deodorant, increase the amount of coconut oil slightly.

This Lavender & Tea Tree Deodorant is a natural and effective addition to your personal care routine, providing your underarms with the soothing and antimicrobial benefits of high-quality essential oils and natural ingredients. Enjoy the fresh and clean feeling.

31. Neroli & Frankincense Anti-Stress Roll-On

This Neroli & Frankincense Anti-Stress Roll-on is designed to help you manage stress and promote relaxation throughout your day. Neroli essential oil offers a calming and uplifting aroma, while frankincense essential oil provides grounding and soothing properties. Combined with a nourishing carrier oil, this roll-on is perfect for on-the-go stress relief.

Ingredients:

- 2 teaspoons of jojoba oil (balances sebum production and is easily absorbed)
- 10 drops of neroli essential oil (calming and uplifting)
- 10 drops of frankincense essential oil (grounding and soothing)
- A 10ml roller bottle
- A small funnel (optional, for easier pouring)

Instructions:

1. **Prepare Your Workspace:**
   - Ensure that your roller bottle and any mixing tools are clean and dry. Sterilizing the bottle by rinsing it with boiling water and letting it air dry can help prevent contamination.
2. **Combine Carrier Oil and Essential Oils:**
   - In a small bowl or directly in the roller bottle, combine 2 teaspoons of jojoba oil with 10 drops of neroli essential oil and 10 drops of frankincense essential oil. Stir or shake well to mix.
3. **Mix Thoroughly:**
   - If mixing in a bowl, stir the mixture thoroughly to ensure the essential oils are evenly distributed. If mixing directly in the roller bottle, cap the bottle and shake well to combine all ingredients.
4. **Transfer and Store:**

- o   If you mixed the ingredients in a bowl, use a small funnel to transfer the mixture into your roller bottle. Cap the bottle tightly.
5. **Label and Store**:
   - o   Label the roller bottle with the contents and date. Store the roll-on in a cool, dark place to preserve the integrity of the oils. The roll-on should be used within six months for the best results.

Application:

- Apply the roll-on to your pulse points (wrists, temples, neck) whenever you feel stressed or need a moment of calm.
- Gently massage the oil into your skin using circular motions.
- Breathe deeply and enjoy the calming and grounding aroma.

Tips:

- Perform a patch test before using the roll-on to ensure you don't have any allergic reactions to the essential oils.
- Customize the blend by adjusting the essential oils to your preference, keeping the total number of drops the same.
- For an added cooling effect, store the roll-on in the refrigerator.
- Use the roll-on as part of your daily self-care routine to promote relaxation and stress relief.

This Neroli & Frankincense Anti-Stress Roll-on is a convenient and effective way to manage stress and promote relaxation throughout your day, providing calming and grounding benefits, enjoy the peace and tranquility.

7. SUMMARY

As you reach the end of this journey through "The Monthly Switch: 31 Essential Oil Recipes to change your Makeup Bag" you have not only discovered the transformative potential of essential oils but also embarked on a path toward a healthier, more natural approach to beauty. The recipes provided in this ebook are designed to harness the pure, potent benefits of essential oils, offering you a range of holistic solutions for your skincare, haircare, and overall well-being.

The world of essential oils is vast and rich with possibilities. These natural elixirs, derived from the essence of plants, offer a safe, effective, and environmentally friendly alternative to conventional beauty products laden with synthetic chemicals. By choosing to create your own cosmetics using high-quality essential oils, you are making a conscious decision to prioritize your health, protect the environment, and support ethical and sustainable practices.

Throughout this ebook, you have learned the importance of selecting high-quality essential oils, understanding their therapeutic properties, and incorporating them into various beauty recipes. Whether you are soothing your skin with a calming lavender and chamomile facial serum, stimulating hair growth with a rosemary and peppermint blend, or indulging in a luxurious rose and geranium body butter, each recipe has been crafted to provide maximum benefits with minimal ingredients.

By embracing natural beauty, you are not only enhancing your appearance but also fostering a deeper connection with nature. The act of creating your own beauty products can be both empowering and meditative, allowing you to take control of what goes on your skin and into your body. This practice encourages mindfulness and self-care, reminding you to take time for yourself and appreciate the simple, natural ingredients that can make a significant difference in your beauty routine.

Moreover, the benefits of natural beauty extend beyond personal care. By opting for homemade, natural cosmetics, you are reducing your environmental footprint. Essential oils and other natural ingredients are biodegradable and less harmful to the planet compared to synthetic chemicals found in many commercial products. Many brands committed to producing pure essential oils also adhere to ethical sourcing and cruelty-free practices, ensuring that your beauty choices are aligned with values of compassion and sustainability.

The recipes provided in this ebook are just the beginning. As you become more familiar with essential oils and their benefits, you can experiment with new combinations and create personalized blends tailored to your specific needs and preferences. The possibilities are endless, and the journey of discovery is ongoing.

Remember, the key to achieving the best results with natural beauty products is consistency and patience. Unlike synthetic products that often promise quick fixes, natural remedies work harmoniously with your body's natural processes, promoting long-term health and beauty. Give your skin and hair time to adjust to these new, nourishing treatments, and you will begin to see and feel the positive changes.

We hope this ebook has inspired you to explore the world of essential oils and natural beauty. By integrating these practices into your daily routine, you are taking an important step toward a more holistic, sustainable, and health-conscious lifestyle. The power of nature is at your fingertips—embrace it, enjoy it, and let it enhance your natural beauty.

Thank you for choosing "The Monthly Switch: 31 Essential Oil Recipes to change your Makeup Bag." May this guide serve as a valuable resource on your journey to natural wellness and beauty. Here's to a beautiful, healthy you, inside and out.

ABOUT THE AUTHOR

Lucy is a dedicated registered nurse, a passionate advocate for preventative healthcare, and an enthusiastic educator on non-toxic living. As a married mother of three, she balances her professional expertise with the joys and challenges of family life.

Her journey into the world of natural wellness began with her commitment to providing the best for her family, seeking out ways to reduce their exposure to harmful chemicals. This passion has led her to share her knowledge and experiences, empowering others to make healthier, more informed choices.

Beyond her professional and educational pursuits, Lucy enjoys expressing her creativity through various projects, singing, and cherishing moments with her loved ones. Her holistic approach to health and wellness is deeply rooted in her belief that a balanced, natural lifestyle can lead to a happier and healthier life for everyone.